INTRO

Health is a fact of life. We can't pretend we don't have it.

Just as our physical health can change - any of us can break a bone or become ill - so can our mental wellbeing.

The mental health organisation Mind reckons that, in any given year, one person in four will have a mental health challenge. In any given week, one in six experiences a common mental health problem such as anxiety or depression.

In other words, not feeling great is common. Sometimes it has a perfectly natural explanation: perhaps something like exam or work worries or even something bigger like losing someone close to you. The important thing is that we notice it and do something about it. This is more important if it keeps happening or happens in situations where there's no obvious explanation.

Living in a Covid-19 world is a new challenge. It has increased isolation, loneliness and everyday stress and anxiety. Some have been bereaved, others are living with the long-term impact of the virus. Some have had treatment for their health issues, including mental health conditions, interrupted.

This booklet will help if you're feeling fine and want to keep it that way or if you're feeling crap and want some positive, effective ways to feel better.

THE 'CAN DO' APPROACH

This booklet is built on five proven, evidence-based ways to wellbeing. They are **CONNECT**, get **ACTIVE**, **NOTICE**, **DISCOVER** (or learn) and **OFFER** (or give). **CAN DO** is just an easy way to remember them.

They're so good that many health professionals now prescribe them. Try to get a good balance of all five - like a healthy diet.

There are over 50 challenges in the booklet, so you're bound to find some you like. The truth is we **CAN DO** a lot to boost our mental wellbeing.

C - Connect   page 5

A - Active   page 7

N - Notice   page 8

D - Discover page 10

O - Offer   page 12

HOW TO USE THIS MANUAL

> If you're feeling good right now, just read through the booklet. Dip in where you fancy and try some of the checks and challenges.

> If you're not feeling great, start with the section 'How Are You?' on page 16.

THE WARNING SIGNS

How do we know if our mental wellbeing is not all it could be? Anger, anxiety and stress often feel like natural reactions. Sometimes we feel them so often, we stop noticing. (Perhaps only noticing them in others.) That doesn't mean they're not having an impact on our mental health.

What rattles our cage varies from person to person. But the warning signs are pretty similar for all of us which means we can learn to recognise them.

> Mood swings or sudden anger at relatives, friends, colleagues or pets

> Low self-esteem - thinking negative things about yourself

> Not sleeping properly (or wanting to sleep all the time)

> Feeling really tired and lacking in energy

> Withdrawing from family and friends - not wanting to see people

> Finding it hard to concentrate and struggling at work

> Poor memory or forgetfulness

> Eating more or less than normal

> Excessive drinking and/or drug use

> Behaving out of character

> Losing interest in things you enjoy

> Unusual experiences, like seeing or hearing things that others don't

> There may also be physical symptoms like headaches, irritable bowel syndrome or aches and pains.

If you're experiencing these, especially more than one, you should probably think about your mental wellbeing.

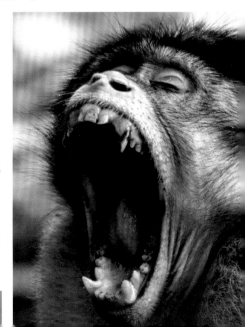

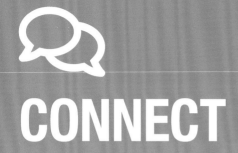

CONNECT

Family, neighbours, workmates... we can take it for granted that we're connected to other people.

But we need to work on those connections and make new ones too. Why? There is good evidence that feeling close to, and valued by, other people boosts mental wellbeing.

It's natural and healthy to want to be on your own occasionally, but we're all different. Levels of contact which feel like too much for one person may make another feel lonely. It's not the amount of contact but how you feel about it. People who feel lonely are at a much higher risk of health problems. The risk to life has been compared to smoking about 15 cigarettes a day.

If you feel lonely, try to take on some of the CONNECT challenges listed below. (Bear in mind any government guidelines on social distancing.) There's no need to get into long conversations unless everybody involved wants to. When it comes to connecting, a little goes a long way.

CHECK: HOW CONNECTED ARE YOU?

> Log your contacts for a week or a month - who do you have contact with? (include family, friends, work) How long and often?

> What's the 'quality' of the time? Is it meaningful to you?

> How could you connect more and connect better?

Challenges...

☐ Talk to someone who you generally text or email.

☐ Call an old friend or relative who you've lost touch with.

☐ Talk to someone new - where you live, at work, in a social setting or shop.

☐ Ask someone you know something about themselves that you don't know.

- [ ] Offer someone a lift or suggest you travel together.

- [ ] Contact someone you have not spoken to for over a year.

- [ ] Turn off your screens and talk to your partner or those you live with. Set a time. Say, half an hour.

- [ ] Try a new activity which is specifically about meeting people. So going jogging or biking doesn't count, but joining a running or cycling club could.

- [ ] Ask someone for help - it could be with anything but we could all use help with something.

- [ ] Talk to people in the street, bus drivers or shop assistants - even if it's only to say 'hello' or 'good morning'.

ANGER: HOW TO TAKE A TIME-OUT

Feeling angry? Might crack? Try some of these to take a time-out:

> Remove yourself from the immediate source of stress if you can (you could say 'I'm going to the bathroom')

> Give yourself a simple manual or mental task to 'distract' your mind

> Change scenery – somewhere peaceful such as a library, church, garden

> Turn off social media, email and mobile phones

> Take a walk

> Breathe deeply from the waist rather than the chest to relax the body (search online for 'diaphragmatic breathing').

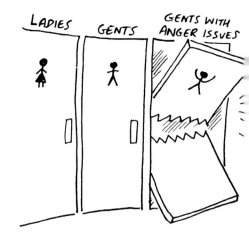

If you're being physically or psychologically violent to a partner or someone you live with, talk to someone. The Respect helpline can help you stop (0808 8024040 or respectphoneline.org.uk). The Men's Advice Line is for men on the receiving end of domestic violence (0808 8010327 or mensadviceline.org.uk).

BE ACTIVE

When we're feeling down, we often can't be bothered to take exercise or be active. But that is the time when we most need it. Taking part in regular physical activity boosts wellbeing.

Try to get active everyday. It doesn't need to be one long session. Every little helps. Three ten-minute walks will do the job. Fifteen minutes of yoga is better than none. Cycling doesn't have to mean lycra, just use your bike as a means of transport. Active DIY or decorating also provides a sense of achievement.

Don't worry about how 'intense' the activity is. (Gardening, for example, is great exercise.) Just find something you enjoy. Take it easy, don't get injured and do it regularly. (If you want to start running, try the Couch to 5K.)

CHECK: HOW ACTIVE ARE YOU?

Monitor your physical activity for a week or a month. What do you do and for how long? A phone app can help, even if it's just to count the steps you walk.

Challenges...

☐ Take the stairs, not the lift.

☐ Get off the train or bus a stop earlier or park the car further away.

☐ Do stretching exercises (try them when you first get up in the morning).

☐ Try an activity (eg. cycling or swimming) that you have not done for a while

☐ Try a new activity that you've never done.

☐ Combine being active with connecting: sport, walking, gardening. (And yes, sex ticks the box.)

☐ Walk every day - set yourself a target. The experts suggest 10,000 steps but 5,000 or less is fine. Simply do it everyday.

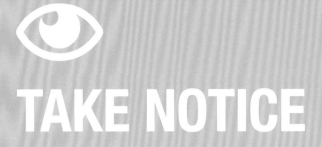

TAKE NOTICE

This is about being aware of what is taking place in the present.

It sounds easy, but the truth is that we're often thinking about the past or fretting about the future, rather than fully participating in the moment we are living. Mobile technology can make this even more difficult.

On the other hand, this is probably the easiest of the five ways to do something about. Just slow down. Engage your senses. Taste what you're eating and drinking. Listen to the sounds around you. Notice the environment you're walking or driving through.

CHECK: ARE YOU TAKING NOTICE?

Monitor your environment for a week or a month.

> How many different types of places do you go to? Is it all urban or do you get out into the green or near water?

> How observant are you? Can you describe your living room or office or local park without going to it?

Challenges...

☐ Turn off your phone for an hour.

☐ Look up at the sky and rooftops, rather than down at the pavement.

☐ Take a different route on a familiar journey.

☐ Go somewhere new for lunch.

☐ Spend more time in parks, forests or at the seaside.

☐ Choose some wildlife (depending on where you live, it might be cats or dogs, birds, bees or butterflies or something more exotic). Watch them for a week. How many? How many different types?

- [ ] On your next walk, find five beautiful things: a cloud formation, a tree, the light, a bird, the leaves, a building, a colour, anything at all - things that please your eye.
- [ ] Plant something or put up a bird box or a window box.
- [ ] Take photos of interesting things - not just selfies.
- [ ] Do some gardening for yourself or someone else - perhaps you can volunteer at a local park?
- [ ] Find some scents you like and inhale them regularly - coffee, favourite herbs, essential oils, your partner's T-shirt or favourite perfume.
- [ ] Listen to music and nothing else - turn off the lights, close your eyes. (Don't fall asleep.)
- [ ] Have a meal or a drink outside. This is an even better idea in a Covid world (though follow social distancing guidelines) but easier said than done in the British weather. Just having a cup of coffee at an open window can be calming (though it depends on the view). Get outside at lunchtime.
- [ ] Try drawing or sketching, pastels or paints.
- [ ] Go to a place near you that you've never been to before - museum, beauty spot, place of worship - and check it out.

NEED SOME 'BREATHING SPACE'?

Learn a three-minute breathing space exercise. This is a simple technique for helping you to stop fretting about whatever's on your mind and get back into the moment. Search 'three-minute breathing space exercise' online.

If you want to take this further, look into mindfulness. If you also want to make it a little more energetic, consider yoga, pilates or tai-chi.

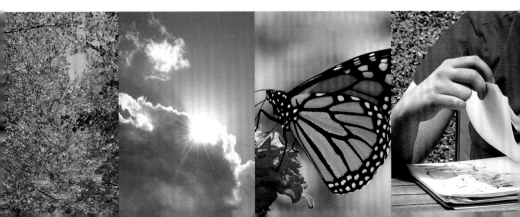

DISCOVER

Learning isn't just something that happens in formal settings like schools or colleges, it is something that continues throughout our lives.

Thinking about it as 'discovery' may help. Learning new things, whatever your age, boosts mental wellbeing and helps protect against diseases like dementia.

CHECK: HOW MUCH ARE YOU LEARNING?

> What have you learned over the last month?

> What have you learned over the last year? Write it down or record it.

> What things would you like to discover or learn about in the future?

Challenges...

- [ ] Read a book - reading is proven to reduce stress, boost concentration, help sleep, aid empathy and connection and strengthen your brain (including against ageing).
- [ ] Sign up for a class.
- [ ] Do some puzzles.
- [ ] Research something you are curious about (eg. your family tree).
- [ ] Take up a language (Duolingo is a popular free app) or a musical instrument.
- [ ] Learn a new practical skill (eg. how to fix your bike).
- [ ] Play a game or sport that you've never played before.
- [ ] Learn to cook some new dishes - got ingredients in your fridge? Search online for recipes that use them.

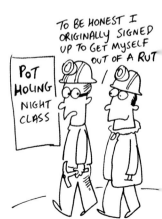

TO BE HONEST I ORIGINALLY SIGNED UP TO GET MYSELF OUT OF A RUT

PoT HOLING NIGHT CLASS

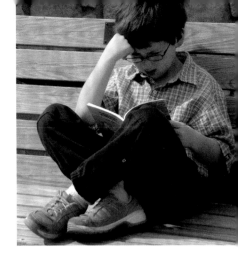

BOOKSHELF

Books, audiobooks, comics, they're all fine. Looking for some reading ideas? Try these:

> a novel by a woman

> a book first published in another country

> a book first published in another century

> a local history book to discover more about the area you live in

> a book about your favourite sport but not your favourite player/team (City fans, read about United).

FOOD AND DRINK

Make sure you're eating properly. There's no room in this booklet to go into detail but you know the basics.

For mental wellbeing, eat regularly, get some protein, keep hydrated, avoid too much caffeine and have your five-a-day of fruit and veg.

Too much sugar is linked to depression. Beat cravings by eating more slowly, drinking water or herbal tea instead and going for a walk (even a short one) after a meal.

Watch out for alcohol. Don't try to make yourself feel better by drinking. It doesn't work. Alcohol is a natural depressant and dehydration afterwards will lower your mood further. If you always have a drink at a particular time (such as after work or in front of the telly), take back control and cut it out. See how you feel.

Challenges...

☐ Keep a food and drink diary for a week. Just seeing it in black and white will help. How healthy is your diet? Where could you make changes to improve it?

☐ Can you cut out added sugar for a week?

☐ Stop drinking for a month.

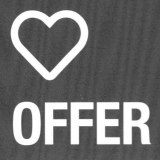

OFFER

Giving something to others doesn't just help them. The evidence is that it helps us too, perhaps even more.

We feel good about what we've done and learn more about the lives of others, which helps us to connect more with people.

CHECK: WHAT ARE YOU OFFERING?

What have you done for others in the past week or month? Include your family and friends as well as any more formal volunteering. Think back on some of those activities, even small ones like making someone a cup of tea. How did they make you and the other person(s) feel?

Challenges:

☐ Volunteer for a charity or community group.

☐ Visit an elderly relative or neighbour.

☐ Do someone a favour.

☐ Offer to help someone with something.

☐ Make eye contact with someone, smile and say thanks.

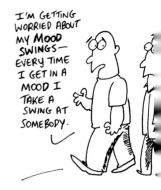

I'M GETTING WORRIED ABOUT MY **MOOD SWINGS** — EVERY TIME I GET IN A MOOD I TAKE A SWING AT SOMEBODY.

GIVE THANKS

What are you grateful for in your life? It's easier to notice the negative things in our lives. But there's a lot of evidence that stopping and thinking of the good things help us as individuals. It makes us feel better. In your diary, phone or wherever, try to record one thing every day that you're grateful for, however small. Perhaps your son took a dirty plate out to the kitchen or your football team's goalie saved a penalty. Perhaps the sun shined.

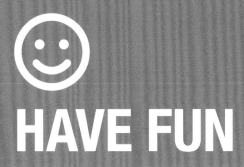

HAVE FUN

If there was a sixth way to wellbeing it would be to have fun. Singing, dancing and laughing are all scientifically proven to boost mood.

Laughing with others rather than at them appears to be best for mental health - presumably because laughing at someone rather than with them often comes from a place of fear.

CHECK: ARE YOU HAVING A LAUGH?

When was the last time you laughed? Keep track for a couple of days.

Challenges:

- [ ] Watch an episode of your favourite comedy programme (could this challenge <u>be</u> any easier?)

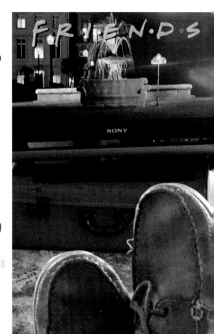

- [ ] Do something you used to enjoy as a kid - build a camp, make Lego, race toy cars. (If you decide to climb trees or go skateboarding, be safe. A visit to A&E is not good for physical or mental health.)

- [ ] Do something creative - paint, write a poem, make a model.

- [ ] Sing - the way we breathe when singing is a natural mood-booster (yes, we're prescribing karaoke for health!)

- [ ] Dance - put your favourite tune on and move.

- [ ] Write - putting down on paper how you feel can help you make sense of it. But write anything you want - fact, fiction, fantasy...

ANYTHING ELSE?

SLEEP

None of these ideas will be as effective as they should be if you're not sleeping properly.

Try to get into a regular night-time routine. Aim for eight hours at roughly the same time every night. (If work and family mean you have no control over when you get up in the morning, it's down to you to go to bed earlier.)

> no screens in the bedroom (includes TV and phones/tablets) or for an hour before bed

> no stimulants, except sex, before bed (no coffee, drugs, vigorous exercise, booze, etc)

> perhaps try some relaxation exercises such as yoga or similar

> or a warm bath

> if thinking about what you need to do keeps you awake, try writing tomorrow's 'To Do' list to clear your head

> reading something light or listening to the radio may relax the mind by distracting it.

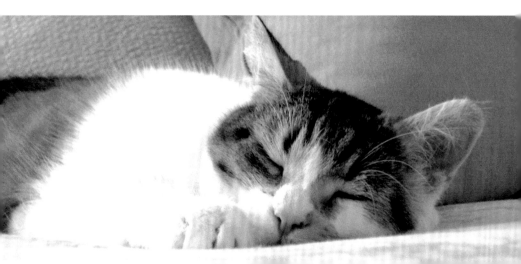

ADDICTION

Drink, drugs, gambling... you can be addicted to pretty much anything.

Symptoms of addiction include depression and anxiety. You may be using your addiction to mask these. Work and relationships are often affected. If you're concerned, ask yourself these questions:

> Do you think about X when you are doing something else and look forward to it?

> Do you feel you need more X each time to get the same enjoyment?

> Have you made efforts to cut back on X?

> Do you do X for longer than intended?

> Have you put X before more important things in life like relationships or work?

> Have you lied to others about your involvement with X?

> Do you use X as a way of escaping from problems or of relieving, for example, feelings of guilt, anxiety or depression?

If you answer yes to some of these, stop X for a month. If that is too difficult, then you have a problem and need to do something about it.

ROUTINE

If you feel like you're losing control, one way to take it back again is to create a clear routine for yourself.

As well as getting up and going to bed at regular times, make a list of what you'll do today. Set small, manageable goals - like tidying up the house for 15 minutes. Take it one task at a time and one day at a time.

Challenges...

☐ Go to bed and get up at the same time for a week. How do you feel?

☐ If someone else is concerned about something you're doing (drinking, gambling, whatever), don't get angry, go through the addiction checklist to make sure.

☐ Make a daily 'done' list - start with three small manageable goals a day.

HOW ARE YOU?

How are you? That question is difficult to answer accurately.

We all say 'fine' if someone asks. The fourteen questions here are widely used to help health professionals go a bit deeper than this. You can use them to help figure out how you're really feeling.

The more honest your answers, the better guide you'll get. (It's only between you and yourself, so be as accurate as you can.)

1. I've been feeling optimistic about the future.

2. I've been feeling useful.

3. I've been feeling relaxed.

4. I've been feeling interested in other people.

5. I've had energy to spare.

6. I've been dealing with problems well.

7. I've been thinking clearly.

8. I've been feeling good about myself.

9. I've been feeling close to other people.

10. I've been feeling confident.

11. I've been able to make up my own mind about things.

12. I've been feeling loved.

13. I've been interested in new things.

14. I've been feeling cheerful.

> **Score all the questions like this:**
>
> a) If you feel like this **NONE** of the time, score **1 point**
> b) if you feel like this **RARELY**, score **2 points**
> c) **SOME** of the time: **3 points**
> d) **OFTEN**: **4 points**
> e) **ALL** of the time: **5 points**

MY SCORES

Date:										
Score:										

Don't get too hung up on the scores. They're most useful for monitoring your mood changes over time. If you score higher in a fortnight than you do today, it suggests your head health is moving in the right direction.

The questions are called the WEMWBS - the Warwick-Edinburgh Mental Wellbeing Scale.

As a rule of thumb:

Under 32 points: your wellbeing score is very low.

32-40 points: your wellbeing score is below average.

40-59 points: your wellbeing score is average.

59-70 points: your wellbeing score is above average.

But, however you score, the challenges in this booklet will help. Read the booklet from the start. Then choose a section that you fancy and dive in. Try the checks and challenges and see how you're feeling in a week and then a fortnight.

TALK

If you score low and still score low a fortnight or month later, you might want to talk to someone. This could be a friend, family member or health professional.

But if you'd prefer someone who doesn't know you, the Samaritans are not just for people who feel suicidal (although they are excellent if you do feel this way). You can talk to their volunteers anonymously about how you're feeling at any time at all by phone (116 123) or by email (jo@samaritans.org).

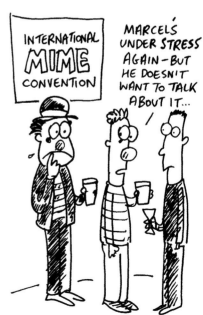

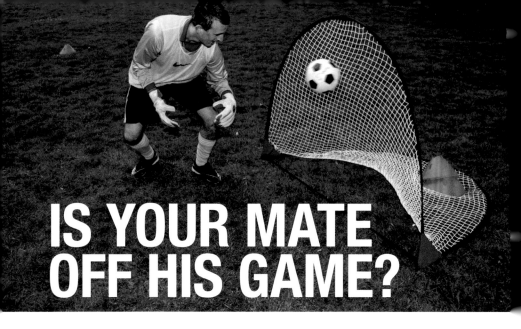

IS YOUR MATE OFF HIS GAME?

As we've seen, every year, one in four of us faces a mental health challenge. That's odds of 3/1, meaning we all know someone affected.

Because we don't really understand mental health problems, sometimes we shy away from people who have them. We pretend we're different, that these things won't affect us. But they do. They hit people just like you.

If we don't tackle our mental health challenges, they can get very serious indeed. The male suicide rate in 2019 was the highest for twenty years. Three out of every four of the people who take their own lives are male.

So, if you think a mate is bottling something up, there's a simple way to make a difference: do something together - car, computer, exercise, garden, walk, DIY, housework. Get him to give you a hand. Feeling wanted makes us all feel better. You don't have to talk seriously (chatting about football is fine), but if you want to, doing something together makes it easier. Open up yourself - if you think he has work issues, maybe talk about your own work. Try to:

> Ask 'How's it going?'

> Keep it real: take it seriously but don't make it a big deal.

> Keep in touch more: text or email.

> Doing stuff is as good as a chat: let your mate see that you know he's still the same person.

> Talk. Swap stories: don't ignore the difficult stuff if it comes up - you don't need to solve it or be an expert, you just need ears.

> Be there: ask if you can do anything. Perhaps, give him this booklet.